I0116304

Diet Fads - Quick Weight Loss Tricks What is the Best Choice for You?

Find a Quick Fix Diet to Suit Your Needs

By Sharon Kingsley

All rights reserved.
This book or parts thereof may not be reproduced, distributed or transmitted in any form by any means—electronic, mechanical, photocopy, recording, or otherwise—without prior written permission of the publisher, except as provided by United Kingdom copyright law.

For permission requests, write to the publisher.
The information contained within this Book is strictly for educational purposes. If you wish to apply ideas contained in this Book, you are taking full responsibility for your actions.

Please check out my other books

Table of Contents

Introduction

There are times in life when we want to look our very best. Of course, you might want to look your very best most of the time, but there are general occasions when this is more important than ever before. We're talking about events such as weddings (either yours or someone else's), vacations, a big party looming on the horizon, that kind of thing.

These types of events require us not only to have our hair done perfectly, make up contoured to perfection, nails immaculate, and eyebrows tweezed to within an inch of their lives, but they also require us to look our slimmest too.

Whether this is wrong or right, it's the truth of the matter. If you're getting married, you want to get into that dress, or into that tuxedo, without feeling extra pounds spilling over the top. If you're heading off on vacation, you want to head to the beach without feeling self-conscious. If you're about to attend a big party or function, you want people to be talking about how fantastic you look, not how you've gained a few pounds.

Whether you're male or female, everyone wants to hit that happy weight. Your happy weight is completely personal to you; it doesn't need to be skinny, it doesn't need to be curvy, it's a weight at which your body settles into a natural plateau, where you can look your best, feel fantastic, and wear whatever you want. The problem is, if you're short on time, e.g. that wedding or vacation is looming large on the horizon, how are you supposed to lose those extra pounds and hit that happy weight on time?

It can be difficult.

Enter the fad diet.

What to Expect from This Book

We need to fill out a slight disclaimer here and now. We do not endorse unhealthy diets. We need to get that out there. What this book is about is using proven weight loss measures on a short-term basis, in order to hit the happy weight, you want achieve.

Fad diets are not meant to be long term deals; they're actually quite unsustainable for the most part! For a quick fix however, a fad diet could be just the ticket you're looking for. The bad news? There are so many out there, it can be hard to figure out which ones are quality, and which ones should be avoiding like the plague.

This book is going to give you the low down on the most popular fad diets out there. Some of these diets can be used in the long term, e.g. the Atkins and the Keto Diet, however there are certain health warnings to all of them. We're going to talk in detail about the warnings, and you should 100% heed this advice!

At the end of the day, the only way to successfully lose weight and keep it off, whilst living a healthy lifestyle, is to make a total lifestyle change. Diets shouldn't be fads, they should be long-term changes to the way we live. What you can do, is use that fad diet to get to where you need to be, and then utilise the healthy eating habits you learn in your long-term life, incorporating exercise too. That is what this book aims to help you to do.

So, whatever the reason for you needing to drop those few extra pounds rather quickly, there is a fad diet out there for you. Why are we calling them 'fad' diets? Well, because most people pick them up and put them down; we mentioned most of them are unsustainable in the long term (except for a select few), hence the name.

Ready to begin?

Chapter 1: What is a Fad Diet?

A fad diet falls into two categories: healthy and unhealthy.

A fad diet become unhealthy when it is used for too long, and when warnings aren't listened to. When a diet is used in the way it is meant to be used, e.g. for a very short time, and in people who have no contraindications to using it, then it can be a very good way to drop weight quickly.

The downside?

You're not really losing weight, most of the time you're losing water, and that means as soon as you begin to eat properly again, that number on the scales is going to dramatically return back to what it was before.

So, are fad diets an illusion? In some ways yes, in some ways no. They do what they say on the tin for the short-term; in the long-term? Questionable.

Many fad diets completely omit major food groups, nutrients, fibre, carbohydrates, vitamins, and minerals. No, that's not good. When this is prolonged, you are running the risk of illness in the long-term. This is the very reason why fad diets are not designed to be used for a long period of time.

The best way to define what a fad diet is, is this - A temporary answer to a problem. If you can use what you have learned during the diet, e.g. you take nutrition seriously and you change your eating behaviour patterns, then you could take something away from the whole experience in the long-term too, provided you ensure you're eating a well-balanced diet, and getting plenty of exercise. The problem is that not many people do that - they simply start to eat normally and notice the scales rising once more. Enter frustration.

Are Fat Diets Dangerous?

We've really answered this question indirectly already. Fad diets *can* be dangerous when they are not used in the right way. If you follow directions, don't use the diet for longer than you should, and if you don't have any health concerns or you're not taking medications, fad diets should be fine. If, however you don't listen to that advice, and you go too far with the diet, yes, they can be very dangerous indeed.

Omitting major food groups, such as carbohydrates or sugars, for a long period of time can take you into serious health issues as you get a little older. This can be irreversible, as the damage will have been done.

Your body's metabolism, e.g. the rate at which it burns food for energy is directly impacted on your diet. When you start to yo-yo between eating habits, you're completely throwing your metabolism up in the air. It basically doesn't know which way to turn. This means it goes into 'starvation mode'. Basically, it thinks you're going to starve, so your body grabs hold of every single calorie and bit of nutrition it can get its hands on. Ironically, this stops you losing weight, because your metabolism slows right down.

On the other hand, when you eat a healthy, balanced diet, the opposite happens.

Most fad diets have a 'scientific' explanation behind them, and they are quite convincing in many cases. Yes, most of these diets have had some kind of research done into them (e.g. the Atkins and the Keto Diet in particular), but results are so mixed, it can be hard to figure out which side of the dangerous and safe level they're on.

Put simply - follow the rules to avoid danger.

Do Fad Diets Work?

They do, yes, but the results aren't meant to last for long. What you are actually losing isn't fat accumulations or inches, it's retained water. This is what goes first whenever you enter into any kind of weight loss programme. This Is the reason why those first few weeks of doing a diet, you're having fantastic losses and it's spurring you on to continue. It's an illusion however, as it's not actual weight that's disappearing.

The flip side of that coin is that by losing retained water, you actually look slimmer. This means you're not as bloated, you'll feel super slim, and your clothes will fit better as a result.

Again, it's an illusion, but it might be one which will serve you for long enough, to get you through that upcoming event you're aiming for.

When you start to eat properly once more; because let's face it, most of these fad diets are completely unrealistic in the long-term, regardless of how committed you are, you'll notice that the weight comes back quite quickly indeed. This is very concerning to those who think that their fad diet is a long-term solution - it's not. This is also the reason why many dieter yo-yo between fad diet to fad diet. The only answer to this conundrum is to realise that fad diets aren't a long-term answer, they're a quick fix. The only long-term answer is choosing overall health and wellbeing over everything else.

When Might a Fad Diet be Useful?

You might think by reading this book so far, that we're trying to complete put you off fad diets altogether. That isn't the aim. All we want you to be aware of is the potential danger, and we want you to go into this endeavour with a realistic mind-frame.

A fad diet can be useful, provided it is followed correctly and for the right length of time, during certain situations in your life, many of which we talked about earlier. If you need to lose weight quickly for a certain event which is coming up, e.g. a wedding or vacation, then a fad diet could give you what you need, but don't expect the results to stick around.

The problem is that sheer number of fad diets which are out there. How are you supposed to know which is the right route for you? Only by arming yourself with the knowledge on each one can you make an informed decision. That is what this book aims to do.

Chapter 2: The Rules of Fad Diets

Before we move into talking about each of the popular fad diets on the market, we need to give you a few rules of the game first of all. This chapter is going to be a quick one, because we've already laid out the facts and what you can expect.

Rules and Time Frames to Bear in Mind

Before choosing any fad diet, any at all, you should heed the following advice:

- Read up on the diet completely, and listen to any advice on how long you can follow the guidelines, in order to avoid damaging your health
- Choose a diet which you feel you can follow without confusing yourself - you need to understand what it is telling you to do properly, and why you're doing it
- Speak to your doctor if you have any health concerns, prior to starting the diet
- Speak to your doctor if you're taking any medications, prior to starting the diet
- Speak to your doctor if you have a strong family history of any medical conditions, prior to starting the diet
- Always drink plenty of water, no matter what fad diet you are following
- If you start to feel unwell whilst you're following the diet, e.g. weak, lethargic, constant headaches, or any other troubling symptoms, stop the diet immediately

A fad diet should not be followed for a long period of time. The amount of time you can safely following a diet depends on the actual diet itself, and what it is doing to your body. By using the words 'short term', we are talking about weeks, and not months! These diets are not sustainable for any longer than that. You will read upon the Keto Diet, Paleo Diet, and the Atkins diet in particular, and they will tell you that this is a total lifestyle change. Yes, in those cases it can be, but those types of diets have phases, which slowly lead you back towards a more 'normal' way of eating. For this reason, those diets need to be followed to the letter, in order to work. Don't worry, we'll talk about the rules of each particular diet as we move through our chapters.

Longevity Vs Short Haul Vs Quick Fix

We've mentioned this already, but let's define each one in turn.

Longevity - The only diet which is suitable in the long term is one which allows you to eat freely in a healthy manner. That means ensuring that your major food groups are satisfied, that you're getting enough vitamins and minerals, and that you're choosing clean foods, rather than processed ones. The Keto Diet, the Atkins Diet, and the Paleo Diet do this to a certain degree, but these all have their own health concerns, which you need to read up on carefully. Most fad diets are not suitable for long-term use.

Short-haul - Some fad diets fit into the short-haul category. This means you're not going to use them for just a week, and it's more likely to be a few weeks or a month. Again, check each diet carefully, but most are suitable for this type of use.

Quick fix - Finally, we have the quick fix. Really, fad diets are best for this type of category. If you have to get into that outfit for your upcoming event, and you're noticing it's a bit tight in certain areas, a fad diet could get rid of that bulging, and allow you to feel svelte for that occasion. After that? The bulge will be back, unfortunately.

Health Concerns and Warnings Related to Fad Diets

Again, this is a really a warning which needs its own sub-section, to draw your attention to its major importance.

Fad diets have health warnings attached to them. If you have any health concerns, if you're taking any medications, of even if you have a family history of a condition, make sure you check things out with your doctor before you begin. If you go ahead and start the diet, you could find that the lack of certain food groups or nutrients exacerbates your original problem, and can cause extra illness.

In addition, you should be on the lookout for any adverse side effects. Yes, many diets have certain side effects; this is down to the transition of eating normally, to eating in a more restricted way. For instance, most diets will cause headaches, but if those headaches are prolonged or severe, that's not normal. In this case, you should stop that diet immediately.

At the end of the day, the old adage 'nothing tastes as good as skinny feels' is a total mistruth. If you're ill, lacking in energy, and feeling completely rubbish, is it really worth it? Keep an eye on how you're feeling whilst you're following the diet, and if something isn't quite right, stop immediately. Remember, one size does not fit all, and you might need to look into a different diet instead.

So, warnings and lectures over, it's time to talk about the most popular fad diets out there, to help you make your own personal choice.

Chapter 3: South Beach Diet

One of the most popular diets out there, and one which has been used by celebrities in glossy magazines, is the South Beach Diet. There was a major boom in interest when this diet first came out, with books on the subject, magazine articles, and enticing weight loss pictures everywhere you turned. It isn't so prominent these days, but it can still be a useful quick fix.

What is The South Beach Diet?

The South Beach Diet was created by a Dr Agatston, a cardiologist, and it is based not he idea of a low carbohydrate intake, with a higher protein and healthy fat substitution. The plus point of this diet is that the carb side of things isn't that strict, so you don't need to buy a carb calculator, or work everything out as you go along.

The plus point of this diet is that one of its primary aims is to help you understand what healthy foods are, versus those which are less than beneficial for your overall health. It doesn't cut out any major nutrient groups, although the lower amount of carbs could be an issue if you don't follow the plan properly. Having said that, the carb counting isn't strict.

The diet was designed to be a long-term food plan, e.g. by lowering the amount of carbs you eat, you're able to lose and the maintain weight in the long-term. The diet also allows you to eat a wide range of different foods, all of which are mostly very healthy and packed with nutrients. The downside is that lowering carbs can have side effects, and needs to be followed with caution if you have diabetes, or a family history of the condition.

Why Does It Work?

The diet claims to allow its followers to eat carbs (in extreme moderation) protein (provided it is of the lean variety, e.g. no bad fats), and healthy fats (no, that doesn't mean pizza). This basically adds up to a fairly nutritious diet, and the education side of it is quite favourable too, as it will help you to differentiate between good fats and bad fats, healthy carbs and unhealthy carbs etc. This is information you can use for life, and to help you maintain a healthy lifestyle afterwards, whether you want to continue following the diet or not. For instance, you'll learn about fruits and vegetables, whole-grains, and why you need fiber in your diet.

The downside is that in order to figure out how many carbs you can eat, and which you can eat, you need to do some mathematics. The diet works with something called the glycemic index, and glycemic load. Foods which are higher on the index, spike your blood sugar, which can cause you to be hungrier quicker. Therefore, you need to think about foods which are lower on the glycemic index. You'll get used to it, the more you practice.

The difference between the South Beach Diet and other low carbohydrate diets is that it isn't as low in carbs as some of the other more restrictive options, which makes it a very attractive option. In this diet, you are generally allowed around 140g of carbs every day. The diet has phases, so you'll eat less carbs at the start, and more as you enter the 'maintenance 'phase. This diet also teaches you the importance of exercise, and basically, the diet is boosted ten-fold by doing some regular exercise, of some kind.

Expected Weight Loss Results

Obviously, the amount of weight you lose is going to be a personal deal, but on average, you can expect to lose around 8-13lb in the first two weeks (phase 1). This weight is most likely to be from the belly, so you will see results quite quickly. As you enter into the second phase, the weight loss slows down, but remains steady, at an average of 1-2lb per week, which is actually the recommended healthy amount for those on a weight loss programme.

Example Meal Plans/Eating Suggestions

To give you the full list of foods you can and can't eat would be exhausting, so let's stick to a general idea. From this, you can see whether this diet is a good option for you.

Phase 1 - You will eat very few carbs in this stage, and you can't drink juice or alcohol. Instead, you can eat lean protein sources, e.g. poultry with no skin, or soy choices. You should also eat plenty of vegetables with a high amount of fiber, dairy which is low fat, and nuts, seeds, and avocados aplenty! This phase lasts for two weeks and is the time you will notice the major weight loss.

Phase 2 - Things get a little easier in phase two. You can now eat some carbs, including whole-grain bread and pasta, brown rice, and you should continue to eat plenty of fruits and vegetables.

Phase 3 - Anything in moderation, provided you don't go over the top! This phase continues on for life.

Warnings

Whilst the South Beach Diet is healthy in principle, it is only really healthy when followed correctly, by those who are able to follow it. Restricting carbs to a high degree for longer than two weeks is dangerous, because by doing this you are actually forcing your body into ketosis (e.g. starvation mode). When this happens, you're burning fat for energy, intends of carbs. A build of ketones (a side product of this process) can cause a lot of side effects. Watch out for any unpleasant side effects which are ongoing.

Anyone with diabetes, or a family history of diabetes should also speak to their doctor beforehand.

Chapter 4: What is Weight Watchers?

Ah, the one we've all heard of! Weight Watchers has been around seemingly forever, and it is a low calorie, low fat diet. Weight Watchers is effective, but it is hard work, because by restricting your fats and calories, you're going to be hungry if you don't follow it correctly!

The plus point of this set is that it is actually nutritionally balanced, provided you follow it as you should. If you try and throw in high fat foods, you're going to find yourself with less to eat for the rest of the day. By teaching you about healthy food choices, you will be less hungry, and you'll notice a steady weight loss. Are the results super-fast? In the first couple of weeks yes, but then it will slow down to a steady 1-2lb per week.

Why Does It Work?

Weight Watchers gives you a certain number of points per day. The amount of points you have depends upon your weight. The more your weight, the more points you start with, and this decreases as your weight decreases too. In order to use up your daily points, all foods and drinks have a points value. As you consume something, you deduct that number of points from your daily allowance. When you reach zero, you're done for the day! You can earn points by doing exercise, which allows you to eat extra foods during that particular day. You cannot carry points over to another day.

Why does it work? Because you're limiting your calories and fats. By doing this, you're producing a calorie deficit, e.g. you're burning more than you're eating. This is going to result in weight loss, albeit steady. You can increase your results with exercise, and in the first few weeks your loss will be higher, basically because you're losing retained water.

The downside of Weight Watchers is the counting of points. You will become super aware of what is in everything you're eating, and that can become a rather mild obsession. Of course, it can also help you to learn about healthy foods and bad foods, teaching you about healthy choices over the long-term.

Is it sustainable? Yes and no. You cannot be expected to count points for the rest of your days, so the sustainability really depends upon how well and how quickly you learn about healthy food choices. From there, you will form habits which should make this diet quite long-term.

Expected Weight Loss Results

Again, it completely depends upon your starting weight and how well you follow the points counting. On average, the first two weeks will show a greater loss, thanks to a loss of retained fluid, but after that you're looking at around 1-2lb per week, or 8lb per month.

Example Meal Plans/Eating Suggestions

The sheer number of things you can eat on Weight Watchers means we cannot give you a list, once again. What you eat depends on the points amount. For instance, if you eat a bar of chocolate, you're going to use around 8 points, and if you're only allowed 18-20 per day, that's not leaving you with much left! On the other hand, if you choose an apple, you might be looking at something like half a point. Can you see how Weight Watchers helps you make healthier choices? Basically, if you don't, then you're going to be hungry, that's a lesson in itself!

A quick idea of a day's meal plan might include:

• Breakfast - Asparagus quiche with no crust
• Lunch - Turkey and brie panini
• Dinner - Slow cooker chicken pot roast
• Snacks - Fruit

Depending upon your points amount permitted, this could take up just one day's amount.

Warnings

There aren't many warnings with Weight Watchers, and if Oprah loves it then surely that's a good thing! Of course, if you have any health concerns, or if you're on any medications/have any conditions, then you should speak to your doctor first. Certain foods need to be consumed by people who have certain conditions, and you need to ensure that you're getting what you need for your overall health and wellbeing.

The biggest warning with Weight Watchers is about making sure you choose healthy options, to avoid being very hungry at the end of the day! If you don't do this, you're going to simply rebel and eat more of the bad things, certainly not resulting in weight loss, and probably more like a gain.

Chapter 5: The Zone Diet

The Zone Diet has been around for years, and whilst it might not have the media space as some of the big hitters, like the Atkins Diet, it has been the diet of choice for many people who want to drop weight fast, whilst attempting to learn about healthy food choices at the same time. Developed more than 30 years ago by a Biochemist in America, Dr Sears, the diet became more popular after the book was published in 1995.

What is The Zone Diet?

The Zone Diet is different from many other fad diets because it does at least attempt to encourage the person following the diet to eat a balanced amount of food, from different food groups, every day. For instance, you will eat a certain amount of fats (healthy, of course), carbohydrates, and proteins in every single meal, and the idea is that you're reducing the amount of inflammation in the body. This is what the Zone Diet is really based around, inflammation reduction. The idea is that by doing that, you lose weight too.

This diet encourages you to eat 40% carbohydrates, 30% protein, and 30% fat at every meal. This fat needs to be monounsaturated, and the protein needs to be totally lean. By doing this, you are encouraging your body to release energy slowly, therefore keeping you fuller for longer, and losing weight as a result.

Why Does It Work?

Inflammation within the body is responsible for many different health concerns and diseases, whilst also being responsible for fast ageing. The idea behind the Zone Diet therefore is that if you reduce the amount of inflammation in the body, you're encouraging your body to burn fat for energy, therefore reducing your excess fat ratio, and increasing your overall health at the same time.

This diet is a easier to follow than it sounds, because it doesn't have phases, unlike the South Beach Diet, for example. It is however supposed to be something you follow for life, and if you don't want to be thinking about percentages and ratios for the rest of your days, you might find it difficult to sustain over the long-term. As a short to medium-term fix however, it could be useful. At first, learning how to manage the diet can be difficult, however.

In order to follow the diet, and therefore get the percentages right, you need to think about two different methods, either the hand-eye method, or the food blocks method. The former is the easier way to begin, and basically means that you use your eyes to determine food portions and ratios on your plate, and your fingers to remind you to eat five times a day, and not to go longer than five hours with food at any one time. You plate is divided into thirds, in order to estimate your food percentages.

The block method is much more complicated, and requires you to calculate percentages and arrange foods into blocks.

The name 'The Zone' comes from the idea that by following the diet, you are forcing your body into an optimum hormonal state, called 'The Zone'. This state allows you to reduce inflammation and lose weight.

Expected Weight Loss Results

The Zone Diet brings about quite variable weight loss results. As with most fad diets, in the first few weeks, the weight loss is more dramatic, and from there is slows down. The difference with the Zone Diet is that there are no phases, so the weight loss is steadier throughout.

On average, a loss of around 4lb in the first week is possible, with 1-2lb per week from there onwards

Example Meal Plans/Eating Suggestions

There are foods which are not allowed on the Zone Diet, and foods which are recommended. We mentioned the ratio between carbs, fats, and proteins, so this is what you should be mainly focusing on. The idea of explaining the 'zoning' of foods at this stage is going to do nothing but confuse you, so we'll stick to the foods you can eat, and the ones you can't for now.

Meals should include lean protein, so lean pork, veal, game, chicken and beef, cooked in good oils, such as canola oil, olive oil, etc. Meals should also have a good portion of vegetables which are low in glycemic index value, such as peppers, tomatoes, mushrooms, chickpeas, and spinach. You can have fruit for dessert, such as apples, plums, and oranges.

We mentioned foods you can't eat, and whilst that is recommended, it's fair to say that nothing is strictly off limits. Basically, you need to remember the idea of moderation. Anything processed is considered to promote inflammation within the body, and that's the whole thing you're trying to avoid with this diet.

Warnings

There are no special warnings to heed with the Zone Diet, which are any different to the other diets we've talked about so far. If you do have any health concerns or conditions, it's always best to check things out with your doctor.

The Zone Diet controls inflammation within the body, and whilst there isn't a huge amount of scientific evidence to back up its claims, the whole vibe around eating healthily and ensuring you get the correct food groups in your diet is heathy regardless of the aim.

Chapter 6: Mediterranean Diet

The Mediterranean Diet is considered by many to be one of the healthiest around. It falls into the 'fad diet' category because it has rules and regulations, and because over time it could be hard to stick to for life. The Mediterranean Diet teaches you about healthy, clean eating, which is never a bad thing, but there are restrictions of foods you cannot eat, if you want to lose weight and maintain momentum.

What is the Mediterranean Diet?

Based around the healthy foods grown and consumed traditionally in the Mediterranean area, this particular diet has been around for a long time. You will no doubt remember the adverts on olive oil a few years ago, claiming that people from this region lived longer because of what they ate. This is what this diet is based around. What you're basically getting is a lot of healthy food, mostly cooked in olive oil and some delicious red wine too. Sounds good so far!

The foods generally consumed include fruit, vegetables, whole-grains, healthy fats, and fish. Anything unhealthy, e.g. processed and fatty, is out. The idea is that by following this diet, you'll lose weight, yes, but you'll also notice a general increase in your health overall, as well as protecting you against various heart-related issues, including high cholesterol.

A lot of research has gone into whether or not the Mediterranean Diet actually works in terms of heart health, and the results are surprisingly positive. In addition, there is a link with reduced cancer risk and a reduced risk of conditions such as Parkinson's and Alzheimer's.

From reading that, you could consider the Mediterranean Diet to be not at all faddy, but that depends upon compliance. If you follow the diet properly, if you vary your foods and if you actually enjoy the fresh produce on offer, then this could be a very successful and healthy way to live your life in the long-term. Does it offer huge weight losses? In the first few weeks yes, due to loss of water, but after that it slows down. Basically, the Mediterranean Diet is more about overall health and wellbeing than anything else, and will help educate you on healthy food choices.

Why Does It Work?

It should be quite obvious why the Mediterranean Diet has yielded fantastic results for many people. Basically, we're talking about making healthy choices and affecting your body as a result. The weight loss is as a result of cutting out processed, fatty foods, and instead replacing them with healthier options, including exercise into the whole deal.

There isn't anything particularly restrictive about the Mediterranean Diet, and there are no phases to consider, which makes it very easy to follow. Once you have a general idea of the things you should be eating, versus the things to avoid, you should find this diet one of the easiest around.

By eating plenty of the good things, e.g. whole-grains, fruits, vegetables, and lean meats, you're affecting your health and wellbeing in a very positive way, without having to calculate points, weights, or glycemic indexes!

Expected Weight Loss Results

The Mediterranean Diet probably isn't going to give you major, drastic results immediately, but you will notice a loss of water in the first couple of weeks, which will show on the scales.

As with most fad diets, this isn't a true weight loss, more of an illusion. If you want a quick fix though, and you want to look towards a healthier future, this it's a great options. After that time, weight loss should steady down to the average of most other diets, e.g. 1-2lb per week. The difference is that you should feel you have more energy and basically feel healthier overall.

Example Meal Plans/Eating Suggestions

Overall, when you follow the Mediterranean Diet you should focus mainly on the following:

- Foods which are derived from plants, e.g. fruits, vegetables, legumes, nuts, and whole-grains
- Eat nuts as snacks, e.g. cashews, almonds, walnuts, and pistachios
- Pack your diet with around 10 servings of fruits and vegetables every day
- Cooking with olive oil and canola oil, and avoiding unhealthy fats, including avoiding butter
- Cutting down on the amount of salt you eat, and instead using spices for flavour
- Fish and poultry dishes should be consumed twice a week or more
- You can have red meat, but use moderation
- You can eat pasta and rice, but go for the whole-grain version

- Drink plenty of water
- You can have red wine in moderation
- Stick to dairy products which are low fat

As you can see, the Mediterranean diet is a super healthy choice, and those who follow it properly, i.e. they like the foods and don't mind omitting the unhealthy things, can easily follow it for life.

Warnings

There aren't any specific warnings related to the Mediterranean Diet. Overall, this is considered to be one of the healthiest around. As with any diet however, if you're switching your eating habits drastically, check things out with your doctor ahead of time.

Chapter 7: Atkins Diet

Everyone has heard of the Atkins Diet; you might not really know what it is, but it had such a moment of fame a decade or two ago, which put it right in the spotlight. The problem is, the spotlight was quite a negative one at the time, and this has forced those behind the diet to modify it slightly, to create a healthier version.

What is The Atkins Diet?

Originally created by a cardiologist, Robert C Atkins, in the 1960s, the diet is a low carbohydrate option, one which pushes forward proteins and fats instead. This is a phased diet, and it has to be followed to the letter in order to see progress, but also in order to avoid poor health. The first phase is by far the most restrictive, and this is the point at which many people give up, or notice side effects. The good news is that after those two weeks, you'll notice dramatic weight loss and the side effects should disappear.

Is it healthy though? The sceptics are on the fence, however the idea is now more about making healthy food choices for life, rather than drastically reducing food in the restrictive first phase.

To summarise it, basically the Atkins diet is about eating a balance of carbohydrates (limited), along with protein and fats. By doing this, you are teaching your body to burn fat for fuel, rather than carbohydrates, hence giving dramatic results at the start. The phases are designed to increase the carbohydrate level back a little throughout the following weeks, before your body reaches a 'happy level', which you will stick to for life. If you deviate from this, you will notice weight gain, because you are pushing your body back to its normal state of burning carbs for fuel, rather than fat.

The most attractive thing for those who follow the Atkins Diet is that there is no restriction on fats, in fact it is to be recommended, as eating more fat gives you more fuel to burn. This doesn't mean you can eat any old fats however, and that is a mistake many people make. It is basically all about avoiding carbs, and you will need to keep a track of these through your days. This will become easier, as you become more au fait with what carb amount is in different foods - many have more than you may realise!

Why Does It Work?

It works because you are forcing your body to burn fat for fuel, rather than carbs. You're restricting the carb amount to a level which means your body simply can't use its usual source, so it has no choice but to use fat instead. Yes, you're eating fat and it's going to use that, but it's also going to use up your existing fat stores, which means dramatic weight and inch loss in the first phase. This isn't a sustainable phase however, and should not be used after the recommended amount of time (usually 2 weeks), because the risk of health problems and increased severity of side effects is much greater.

The Atkins Diet isn't easy; it requires a lot of will power and dedication, but it is a totally new take on what is considered to be healthy. Many doctors do not consider this diet to be healthy at all, and when you consider that the Atkins people don't necessarily recommend you need to exercise, that says a lot. It does however acknowledge that exercise will help to boost results however.

There are three phases with this diet, and we'll talk about what you can eat in a moment. The first phase is the most restrictive, as we have mentioned. In this phase, it is vital that you eat enough fat and protein to sustain your energy levels, as this is the point at which carbs are scarce. It's important to stick to the rules here, because one deviation in carbs will switch your body back to the other method of burning for fuel.

The second phase introduces carbs a little at a time, however they are still quite badly restricted. Whilst not as hard-going as the first phase, this second phase is still relatively difficult, especially for those who love their breads, pizzas, and pastas!

The third stage is your final maintenance phase. At this point, you will understand your body's happy carb amount. This is the amount at which you can consume carbs without putting on or losing weight. You'll stick to this for life, in order to maintain your results.

There are various phase differences, as the Atkins is always evolving and changing, and there are various takes on it too. This is the simplified version.

Expected Weight Loss Results

Whilst doctors might not advocate the Atkins for overall health, there is no denying that this is a diet you will lose weight on quite quickly. Of course, this is because you are restricting yourself quite severely for the first two weeks. It depends how much weight you have to lose, and your overall size to start with, but it isn't unusual to lose around 15lb in the first phase of the diet.

The weight loss doesn't stop in the second phase, but it will slow down slightly, to around 2-3lb per week, depending upon the person. The final stage is about maintenance, so weight loss shouldn't occur during this time.

Example Meal Plans/Eating Suggestions

We've mentioned that the first phase is the hardest, and this is also when you will notice large weight losses, albeit a lot of it via loss of water. To give you more of an idea of how restrictive this first phase is, and what you might be able to eat, this is an example of one day:

- Breakfast - Scrambled eggs with cheddar cheese
- Lunch - Chicken salad with bacon and avocado
- Dinner - Salmon steak with salad and asparagus
- Drinks - You can have water, herbal teas, coffee, tea, or diet soda drinks
- Snacks - No more than two per day, including celery with cheese, or a Atkins snack product

You can see the low carb level in that sample, i.e. no bread, no pasta, no potatoes. The protein and fat element is vital in this first phase, otherwise you're going to have zero energy, a huge amount of side effects, and you're running the risk of illness.

As you move into the second phase, you can start to reintroduce carbs but only very slightly.

Warnings

Where do we start?!

The Atkins Diet is successful, there's no denying that, and over time there is some argument to suggest that switching your diet to this lower carb version, can actually bring some health benefits, such as a greater level of energy. However, it is almost guaranteed that during the first phase you will notice side effects, typically including:

• Headaches
• Dizziness
• Lethargy and lack of energy/weakness
• Constipation
• Muscle aches and pains
• Bad breath
• A lack of focus

These side effects are mainly due to the fact that by restricting your carbs, you are forcing your body into ketosis, something we talked about with the South Beach Diet earlier on.

The almost guaranteed drastic weight loss is what attracts most people to the Atkins Diet, as well as the high fat content. Having said that, this isn't a diet which everyone can follow, and if you have any health concerns at all, especially if you have kidney issues, you are pregnant or breast-feeding, or you have diabetic issues, then you should not follow the diet. If you are currently taking any medications, speak to your doctor first, as certain medications, like diuretics, insulin, or diabetic drugs, can interact with the diet overall.

Chapter 8: Paleo Diet

The Paleo Diet is another of the more famous fad diets around, and it is one which is actually based on prehistoric eating habits.

If you've ever wanted to be a caveman or cavewoman, perhaps this is the diet for you!

The Paleo Diet is however considered to be quite restrictive, although successful for dramatic weight loses. Again, this is not a diet you should take lightly, as it is very restrictive, and for that reason, not very sustainable in the long-term.

What is The Paleo Diet?

You might hear the Paleo Diet named as the Paleolithic Diet, the Stone Age Diet, or the Caveman Diet, but it's all much the same thing. Basically, this diet is based on the way people would have eaten during Paleolithic times, e.g. around 2.5 million years ago. From that description alone, you can understand that restrictive is the word here!

The diet's main focus is around what could be gathered from the land during those times, e.g. as a hunter-gatherer.

The idea is that by changing the way we eat, e.g. returning back to the early days, we're actually becoming more in line with what humans were 'supposed' to eat. Basically, what we're eating now isn't what we were ever supposed to eat, according to this diet. The farming methods we use these days are not matched to the human body's original genetics, and by returning back to those types of foods, we're realigning ourselves.

Of course, the diet works because it's healthy, and it encourages healthier food choices, but it is quite restrictive and therefore probably not stainable for most people in the long-term. The difference between this diet and other similar options is that the Paleo Diet cuts out legumes and whole-grains, a staple in other diets. There is also a lack of dairy products in the Paleo Diet, which are considered to be good protein and calcium sources in most other commercial diets. Instead, you are looking at products which are typically more expensive to buy, such as grass-fed meats, nuts, and wild game products.

Why Does It Work?

The Paleo Diet does work, there is no arguing that fact, but the theory behind it all baffles some. The idea that the diet works because it realigns us with how we were supposed to eat and how we were supposed to farm our foods from the land isn't in line with what many researchers believe to be true, however the diet does encourage healthy food choices, and that in itself is the reason why this diet has some great weight loss and health results.

The problem is, by cutting out whole-grains and dairy products, you're cutting out good fiber and calcium sources, so it is vital that you get your intake of these vital nutrients from other foods. The restrictive nature of the Paleo is a concern for many, despite the fact that the weight loss results are hard to argue with.

You're also completely cutting out processed foods with this diet, and we all know that processed, high fat foods are not good for your overall health and wellbeing, especially for your heart's health too. For that reason, there is a link between the Paleo Diet and overall wellness.

Expected Weight Loss Results

Again, this totally depends upon the person involved, but weight loss on the Paleo Diet is dramatic during the first few weeks, and then slows down, typically. Again, the first week you will certainly lose retained water, which will show drastically on the scales, and after that it will level out to around 2lb per week. The first show of loss could be up to 5lb.

Example Meal Plans/Eating Suggestions

The good thing about the Paleo Diet is that there are no phases to follow, no counting, and no zone control, it's all about a list of foods you can eat, and a list of those you can't. For that reason, the Paleo is quite simple.

Basically, you should eat the following:

• Vegetables
• Fruits
• Seeds
• Nuts
• Meats which are totally lean, grass-fed, or wild game
• Fish, including salmon and mackerel
• Olive oil

On the flip-side, you should avoid the following:

• Any type of grain, e.g. wheat, barley, oats

- Legumes of any type
- Dairy products
- Salt
- Processed foods
- Potatoes
- Refined sugar

Can you see how restrictive that is? For that reason, many assume the Paleo Diet to be not the best choice in the long-term.

Warnings

By switching to the Paleo Diet, you are making major dietary changes, so you should always check with your doctor first. This could come as a shock to your system! Despite that, you are making healthy food choices with the Paleo Diet, albeit restricting your choices quite drastically.

As with any diet, it's about checking things out first, but this is a diet you need to be super dedicated to, without any deviation from the list of dos and don'ts.

Chapter 9: Volumetrics

If you have time to cook, and you're ready to change your lifestyle from unhealthy, to healthy, the volumetric way of life could be for you.

Volumetrics basically aims to help you quit yo yo dieting, e.g. jumping from diet to diet, or from dieting to eating normally, or more than normal. We know that yo yo dieting isn't healthy, as it confuses your body completely. Volumetrics attempts to change that by teaching you about healthy foods, the art of home cooking, and also incorporating regular exercise, for a long-term, healthy way of life.

What is Volumetrics?

Volumetrics was designed by Dr Barbara Rolls, and it focuses on the density of foods, e.g. how many calories they contain. If you can focus on this, reducing the number of calories you eat, and by eating foods which keep you fuller for longer, you're creating that calorie deficit needed for weight loss, but you're also aiming towards a healthier lifestyle overall.

This diet revolves around foods which are low in energy density, e.g. low calorie, but high in water. This means fruits, vegetables, and whole-grains. Good foods, healthy foods. Is it restrictive? In some cases, yes, because you can't cheat and expect to lose weight.

The idea is that by sticking with these low-density foods, you're not going to be as hungry as quickly, you're not going to have the cravings which so often plague dieters, and you're going to be fuller for longer. This all hinges on you sticking to the calorie intake amount, and not going under or over it. As such, there are no foods which are off limit, but a little like Weight Watchers, if you eat something bad, you're stuck for the rest of the day.

In order to get the best meals out of this diet, you need to cook them yourself, because takeaways and ready meals are high in calories, and that's something you're trying to avoid. There is no downside to this however, as learning how to cook is a skill, and you're getting more nutrients as a result! If you don't have the time to cook, that could be an issue for you in terms of this diet.

Taking everything into account, volumetrics isn't really a fad diet per se, it's about knowing the good things to eat, and knowing what to avoid or use in moderation. That's good health sense at the end of the day, and the emphasis on exercise is also a good point. In terms of weight loss however, you're going to have a big loss at the start, because of excess water, and that could be a good starting point, if you need to lose weight quickly.

Why Does It Work?

Volumetrics works because it creates a calorie deficit, e.g. you're eating less calories than you're burning. That's the simple sense to it, and that's probably as basic as a diet can get. The good side is that you will learn to make healthier food choices, and there is no risk to your health, because you're getting all the nutrients you need with this diet/healthy eating plan for life.

You will learn to have treats in moderation, because you will understand that if you eat something high in calories, the rest of your day is going to be fuelled by nothing else but hunger. In that case, you could very easily compare this to Weight Watchers, but it is an easier version because there are no points to count.

Expected Weight Loss Results

It's likely that you will have a big loss in the first week or two, as you're shedding excess water. After that you will slow down to a sustainable 1-2lb per week, and it is thought that this will continue for as long as you follow the diet. The idea is that after that you'll understand about healthy food choice and bad habits, and be able to maintain your loss.

Example Meal Plans/Eating Suggestions

There is no food banned on Volumetrics, but by being aware of the foods which have that low density, means you know what you can eat more of. Again, home cooking is key in this regard, because you can make some seriously delicious and filling meals out of the permitted foods.

Low density foods include:

• Fresh vegetables
• Fresh fruits
• Low fat dairy products
• Whole-grains
• Legumes, especially beans
• Lean meats

You don't need to count much for this diet, but you should keep an eye on the calorie intake you're consuming for the first few weeks, until you begin to understand the amounts in various foods.

Warnings

To be honest, there really aren't any major warnings when it comes to volumetrics. Provided you stick to the foods and create delicious meals, keeping your exercise level up, then you're actually promoting overall health and wellbeing. Having said that, remember to check things out with your doctor if you have any health concerns, before making any dietary changes.

Chapter 10: Raw Food Diet

Yes, you read that right - raw food.

The Raw Food Diet isn't a new thing, and it has been in existence since as far back as the 1800s! Having said that, over the last few years there has definitely been an increase in interest, mainly due to celebrities taking up on the challenge. The idea is that raw food is better for you, because cooking takes away a lot of the nutrients in various ingredients. On the other side of the argument, many doctors argue this isn't the case, and that eating just raw food can actually cause health issues.

You might hear this diet called by other names, such as raw veganism or raw foodism, but it is the same thing.

What is the Raw Food Diet?

In order for a food to be suitable for this diet, it must not have been cooked, e.g. not been subject to heat which is over 48 degrees C. It can't be refined, it can't have been treated with anything false, such as a pesticide, and it can't have been pasteurised. It basically needs to be as fresh, natural, and organic as it is possible to be.

You cannot cook any food, but you can bend it, juice it, soak, sprout, or dehydrate it instead. By the general description, you will understand that this food does not contain any meat, and instead sticks to things which are found on plants and trees, seeds, nuts, fruits, and vegetables. It is possible to add raw fish into the mix, but this should be done with caution. You therefore need to eat 75% raw food in your daily intake, nothing less.

Whilst you can understand the theory behind the diet, studies have shown that raw food isn't really any healthier than cooked food. Yes, cooking can reduce the amount of nutrients in some foods, but it can increase the amount in some others. Cooking also destroys bacteria, which isn't the case when it is raw.

Overall, this diet is very hard to follow for most people, but it is going to give you big weight loss results in the first week or so; after that, it will probably become quite unsustainable.

Why Does It Work?

The Raw Food Diet works, we can't deny that fact. It works because you are drastically cutting down on your calorie intake by eating the foods which are raw, e.g. fruits, vegetables, seeds, etc. Many people believe that by sticking to this diet, you will notice not only weight loss, but also better energy levels, and improved health, but this is to be proven. Of course, you are reducing your impact on the environment, and that's a certainty.

The problem is that when you switch to this rather drastically low calorie diet, you may find it almost impossible to stick to, and you may not be able to meet your minimum calorie amounts for good health. Not everyone loves the foods on the list, and the cravings are likely to be rather severe at first.

Yes, fruits and vegetables are very healthy, and to be encouraged as part of any diet, but when eaten alone, they don't really have enough calories to keep you going through the day, and certainly not enough protein either. In addition, you're not cooking the foods, which could make digestion difficult.

Expected Weight Loss Results

Weight loss on the Raw Food Diet is guaranteed and quite drastic at first. The reason we can't comment past that point is that most people don't stick to it, due to the restrictive nature of the eating plan. The first week or two is likely to see losses, on average, of up to 14lb.

Example Meal Plans/Eating Suggestions

We're probably not painting the greatest picture of this diet, but that's because it is such a difficult one to follow for most people. Some people may find it fantastic, but for the majority of people, the lack of meat and regular carbs, e.g. pasta and bread, is going to be a huge challenge.

There is no counting of much on this diet, simply a list of foods to eat and those to avoid. The only rule is that at least 75% of your daily food should be raw.

Foods you can eat:

- Fruits and vegetables
- Nuts and seeds
- Grains
- Legumes - should be soaked and sprouted first
- Dried fruits
- Dried meats
- Raw nut butter
- Milks derived from nuts
- Cold pressed coconut oil
- Kimchi
- Sauerkraut

- Seaweed
- Spouts
- Raw fish or raw meat (optional)
- Raw dairy, including eggs (optional)

Foods you should avoid:

- Anything cooked, including meats, grains, vegetables, or fruits
- Anything baked
- Anything roasted, e.g. seeds or nuts
- Oils which are refined
- Salt
- Sugar
- Flour
- Dairy which has been pasteurised
- Juices which have been pasteurised
- Tea
- Coffee
- Alcohol
- Pasta
- Potato products
- Anything which is processed

Warnings

This diet is a very restrictive one, and is certainly not for everyone, and probably not at all sustainable for most people. For a quick fix however, it could be a good option, provided you pay heed to checking things out with your doctor first.

A lot of studies have gone into this type of diet and most of them have shown that weight whilst loss is quite drastic, most people have some kind of vitamin deficiency to go alongside it. Over time, bone mass density could be very low, alongside many other detrimental health issues. For that reason, proceed with caution.

Chapter 11: Macrobiotic Diet

Made mainstream by the likes of Gwyneth Paltrow, the Macrobiotic Diet has been around since the 1920s, and actually came from Japan. A philosopher, George Ohsawa, decided that eating a healthy diet, in the simplest of ways, meant that not only would the body thrive and be ultra-healthy on the inside, but that we could also live in total harmony with the world around us, aligned with nature. In addition, Ohsawa believed that the Macrobiotic Diet could cure cancer, however this has never been proven.

What is the Macrobiotic Diet?

The Macrobiotic Diet is completely natural, i.e. nothing false or processed passes the lips. In addition, you could name this diet as a vegan option, as there are no meats eaten, and no dairy products either. Having said that, some people do choose to supplement the diet with fish and meat, but only organic in nature.

The Macrobiotic Diet works alongside the macrobiotic lifestyle, and this means you need to be extremely strict and vigilant about what you eat, what you don't wat, and how you cook it all. Those who take this diet super-seriously often enlist the help of a Macrobiotic Practitioner, who can help create a bespoke plan, based on age, location, lifestyle, etc.

The diet generally consists of foods which are found by foraging, e.g. natural foods, such as barley, oats, buckwheat, and brown rice, as well as anything fruit and vegetable-wise, which has been grown organically. You can also have chick peas, lentils, seaweed, ad fermented soy to add bulk to the diet.

The Macrobiotic Diet teaches you to only eat when you are hungry, and to chew your food until it is literally like water. This ensures good digestion, but also helps you to appreciate the food you have before you. No processed foods are allowed, and nothing which contains anything added in, e.g. preservatives or added sugars. You also can't take supplements or vitamins, as the diet suggests that you should get your entire nutritional intake from your diet alone.

It's also about how you cook your food, and how you prepare it. Everything has to be natural, so you need to store your food in containers which are made of natural products, e.g. wood, glass, or ceramics. You shouldn't cook with electricity, and microwaves are a big no no. Your food should be chopped and prepared in a room without noise and without clutter, and any water you drink should also be purified. In addition to only eating when you're hungry, you should only drink water when you're thirsty, and not otherwise.

If you choose to use a Macrobiotic Practitioner to work alongside your dietary efforts (taking it away from the fad diet to a certain extent), he or she will advise about natural exercises, natural healing, meditation, and advice on how to cook in the macrobiotic way.

Why Does It Work?

The Macrobiotic Diet does work in terms of weight loss, because you're cutting out anything which causes you to gain weight, and you're basically going vegan. The drastic change in your diet is going to result in quite a large weight loss in the first week especially, again down to water loss, and after that you are probably going to see further losses too, but is it sustainable? If you want to go vegan and if you're serious about the environment and being more conscious in that regard, then it could be an option for you, but there are many warnings which work alongside this diet, and we'll cover those shortly.

The Macrobiotic Diet needs to be followed carefully, and you shouldn't be extremely strict with it, because you're going to shock your system from the get go! You should also avoid going to extremes with it, as this diet isn't an easy one to follow and will certainly result in cravings and hunger, until you get used to it at least.

Basically, the reason this diet works in terms of weight loss is because you're upping your fruit and vegetable intake, and you're cutting down on the amount salt, sugar, and fat you eat.

Expected Weight Loss Results

As we just mentioned, the drastic change to your diet is likely to result in a big loss at first, so you could be looking up to around 8lb in the first two weeks, on average. After that, your body is likely to go into what it perceives to be 'starvation mode', and you might find it hard to lose weight for a while. You will generally plateau to around 2lb per week, but most people who aren't 100% committed to the diet will not get to this point, and will simply give up.

Example Meal Plans/Eating Suggestions

The Macrobiotic Diet is a very restrictive one, and if you're a fan of anything carb-related, like bread and pizza, you're going to be miserable, that's for sure! There is a massive list of the foods you can't eat, and that includes anything processed, or anything which has added salts or sugars thrown in too. To make it easier, let's focus on the things you can eat, and give you a general list.

- Whole-grains, which must be organic. These include barley, oats, buckwheat, and brown rice
- Organic fruits and vegetables, locally grown if at all possible
- Soups, which can be made with vegetables
- Seaweed
- Beans
- Chickpeas
- Lentils
- Miso (fermented soy)
- Nuts
- Seeds
- Pickled vegetables (in moderation)
- Organic meat may be eaten if you choose to do so, but only in small amounts
- Organic fish, again if you choose to do so, but small amounts only

Warnings

This diet sounds restrictive, and that's because it is. Many people don't get past the first week or two, which is fine for the fad side of things, and fine for those who want to lose weight quickly, but your weight is going to go back on pretty quick afterwards.

The Macrobiotic Diet, when followed to the letter, doesn't have any meat or dairy in it. Some people choose to have a little organic meat, but that is your choice entirely. The lack of dairy and meat can mean you're missing out on vital nutrients, and your calorie intake is likely to be much lower than what you really need. Yes, this is going to mean weight loss.

Diets such as this should be followed very carefully and only in moderation. Anyone who has any health issues needs to discuss things with their doctor first, and they will almost certainly be advised not to go down this route.

In addition to all of this, the Macrobiotic Diet is not a cheap one to follow. Foods need to be organically sourced and locally grown, making it a difficult option for anyone on a budget.

Chapter 12: NutriSystem

NutriSystem is a 28 day weight loss plan, making it the ultimate short-term fad diet choice. The downside? It costs money.

NutriSystem basically aims to make life easy when you're trying to lose weight. The reason for this is that you don't have to cook anything, and you simply order your meals from the company, and they're shipped to your door every single day. For busy people, this is the ultimate in total convenience.

What is NutriSystem?

NutriSystem is a company, and as we just mentioned, your food will come from the company themselves. This means that you don't have to worry about creating a balanced diet, and you don't need to be concerned about not getting the vitamins and minerals you need. The diet is already counted and nutritionally verified. No need to count points, carbs, calories, nothing. Portion sizes are also already worked out. Of course, you can only eat the foods which are delivered to you, although snacks of fruits and vegetables are permitted in moderation.

The system means that you eat a breakfast, a lunch, a dinner, and a dessert, which are all from the company themselves. The foods are balanced to give you carbs, protein, and fats in the right amount, whilst utilising something called 'smart carbs' which don't give you a blood sugar spike, like some other carbs can. The problem is that you won't be eating anything which is high in GI (glycemic index), and this includes the foods we mostly love, such as white bread, rice, etc.).

Having your food already prepared and delivered to your door might sound great in practice, but the problem with this diet is that it is expensive, you are actively discouraged from eating out, and you cannot drink alcohol for the 28 days you're following the plan.

You do get to choose what you eat from the menu which NutriSystem will send you, and there are a few different plans to choose from, with around 150 different meal choices on offer. There are also plans for men or women in particular, anyone over 60 years of age, vegetarians, and those who suffer with diabetes. All of this means that you don't need to cook, you simply need to heat meals up. If you need to add any foods to the meals, e.g. occasionally you might need to add vegetables, this is going to be adding to the cost, but only marginally.

Why Does It Work?

Everything is already counted out for you in terms of nutrition and calories, so there is less chance of an error, and less chance of a cheat meal being thrown in at some point. This is basically down to the fact you're paying a fair amount of money already for the meals to be delivered to your door. You're also actively encouraged to do around half an hour's exercise every day, to encourage your weight loss further.

Meals are designed to be low in sodium count, as well as containing lean protein sources, smart carbs (as we just mentioned), and plenty of fiber, through many whole-grain ingredients.

Overall, this means that you are getting what you need for health, whilst losing weight at a steady pace. The problem comes when the diet is over, after your 28 days are up, and you have to transition back to cooking for yourself. Many people find that once the convenience is over, the weight starts to creep back on.

Expected Weight Loss Results

NutriSystem isn't expected to give you drastic weight loss results, but in the first week you may notice a larger drop, because of that excess water you're losing. The overall aims is for around 1-2lb per week, however there is a specific programme you can sign up for, called Lean 13. This should give you a loss of around 13lb in a month, on average, as well as many inches lost too.

Example Meal Plans/Eating Suggestions

We can't really give you a list of the foods you can and can't eat, or any meal plan suggestions here, because it completely depends upon the meal choice you opt for from the menu you're given. You do need to eat a breakfast, lunch, dinner, and dessert from the product range, and you can have fruits and vegetables as snacks. No alcohol is allowed, and you should drink plenty of water throughout the day.

A few examples of the meals on offer through the package include oatmeal, muffins and pancakes for breakfast, tacos, chicken and pasta, or soup for lunch or dinner, and you could have a brownie or a cookie as a dessert. These are specifically balanced versions of these foods however, and not the regular ones you are probably used to.

Warnings

As with any diet, you should talk to your doctor before you begin. NutriSystem isn't recommended for pregnant women, anyone who suffers with kidney disease, or anyone who has specific allergies. In addition, anyone under 14 years of age isn't recommended to take part in the diet.

The major downside with the NutriSystem is that you need to sign up for a month and pay up front. This makes this diet quite expensive as a fad choice, and after the pre-packed meals stop being delivered, you might find it hard to transition towards healthy eating, as you haven't had the experience of learning about healthy food choices yourself.

Chapter 13: Keto Diet

The Keto Diet, or the Ketogenic Diet, to give it its complete name, is one of the most popular around, and one you will almost certainly have heard of. The Keto Diet is a low carbohydrate, high fat diet, which forces your body into ketosis, in order to switch from burning carbohydrates for fuel, to burning fat instead.

There are phases to this diet, and in the first phase you are almost guaranteed to have large losses, which will even out as you move into the second phase.

What is the Keto Diet?

The Keto Diet is very popular and it is considered to be a lifestyle choice, not a diet which you dip in and out of from time to time. The reason that you should stick with it, rather than yo yo-ing away, is because you are changing the way your body burns food for fuel, and by going from one to another, you're confusing your system, and increasing the risk of side effects.

On the plus side, when followed correctly, the Keto Diet is very successful at losing large amounts of weight, and also teaches you about healthy food choices, and clean foods. You will eat as much organic as you can on this diet, and you will avoid any type of food which has had anything false added to it. For instance your meat will be grain fed, and your fish will be farmed in a way which avoids any mercury contamination.

The problem with the Keto Diet is that you need to learn about the list of foods you can eat, the foods you can't eat, and the foods you can only enjoy in moderation.

You also need to be able to count net carbs, to ensure that you don't go over your allowed amount during each phase. As you would expect, the first phase is the most restrictive, but this is also the time you are going to lose the most weight. The second phase allows you to add in a few more carbs and other foods, and the third stage is the point you will remain in, e.g. your happy carb amount. From this description, you could argue that the Keto Diet is very similar to the Atkins Diet, but the Keto Diet has a greater emphasis on the clean food side of things.

Your daily intake of food, once you reach the maintenance phase, should be around 5% carbs, 25% protein amount, and 70% fats. As you can see, that is quite high in fat and extremely low in carbs. For that reason, anyone who has any health concerns should speak to a doctor before even considering following this diet.

Why Does It Work?

As with most high fat, low carb diets, the Keto Diet forces your body into ketosis, a state which changes the way your body burns food for fuel. In this state, you will burn fat for energy, rather than carbs, because your body can't get enough carbs to do what it needs to do. This means your existing fat stores will disappear quite quickly, and you will then burn from what you're eating, resulting in further weight loss, and no gains.

The biggest pull for the Keto Diet, aside from the weight loss, is that the diet promises no cravings and no hunger, after the first phase is over.

The reason it works is that fat burning switch being on, however there is concern amongst healthcare professionals about whether ketosis over a long period of time, and in terms of limiting carbohydrates to such a great degree.

Despite all of this, we can't argue with the fact that the Keto Diet works, and it also teaches you about healthy choices and the importance of going organic and 'clean' with your foods.

Expected Weight Loss Results

Keto Diet weight loss expectations vary wildly, and it completely depends upon your weight at the start. The first phase is going to see results of up to 13lb on average, but most of that could be water you're losing. You will also be drinking a lot of water in this phase, which is going to make you feel slimmer, and show on the sales as a false loss.

As you enter the second stage, weight loss will continue, but it will slow to a more expected rate of around 2-3lb on average. Your maintenance phase shouldn't result in any weight loss, but it shouldn't result in gains either.

Example Meal Plans/Eating Suggestions

The foods you can eat on the Keto Diet is long, and the foods you can't eat, as well as the ones you can have in moderation, are equally as long! Meal planning is vital with this diet, to stop you going over your carb amount and to ensure that you stay on target. This isn't a diet you can 'wing', and you need to be very present in the process.

To give you an idea of what you can expect to be eating during that restrictive first phase, a day's diet plan could look something like this:

- Breakfast - A square of spinach and sausage frittata and a coffee made with heavy cream
- Lunch - Egg salad with bacon (no bread!)
- Dinner - Rotisserie chicken and salad. You could also have a cauliflower gratin on the side
- Snacks - Half an avocado with salt, raw almonds

There are so many meal suggestions on the Internet for the Keto Diet that you will find very innovative ways to use your limited first phase ingredients.

It is vital that you get your protein in every day, as well as a good amount of fat. If you don't do this, you're going to be staring illness in the face. We should also mention that during that first phase, you're likely to suffer from side effects, as your body gets used to ketosis. This is also when the famous 'keto flu' might kick in, which mimics the effects of the common illness. Don't worry however, it's very temporary.

Warnings

Any low carb diet should be approached with caution, but if you have any health concerns or conditions, or if you're taking any regular medications, talk to your doctor first. There are also many side effects to take into account with the first phase of this diet, including tiredness, lack of energy, muscle cramps, headaches, cravings (first phase only), and needing to pee quite a lot.

Chapter 14: Copenhagen Diet

Put simply, if you want drastic results, and you want to make yourself miserable for 13 days, the Copenhagen Diet might be the fad diet you're looking for. We do need to do a disclaimer here however, as this is an extremely low calorie diet, and anyone following it needs to be in tip top health, and needs to follow it very carefully indeed.

Also, known widely as the Royal Danish Hospital Diet, the Copenhagen Diet lasts for 13 days, and it is impossible to follow it for any longer than that; most people don't manage the 13 days in the first place.

What is the Copenhagen Diet?

The Copenhagen Diet is not one which anyone would choose to follow for fun, let's put it that way. The diet restricts your daily calorie amount to just 600 per day. That sounds a lot, but when you put it into perspective, and realise that the typical amount for a man is 2500 per day, and a woman needs 2000 per day, you can see how drastic this diet is.

Of course, there has to be an incentive, and that is that the diet promises lose of up to 22lb during the 13 days. Does it stay off? No. As soon as you stop the diet, it is very likely to come back on, and a lot of what you're losing is simply water. The fact you are severely restricting your calorie intake also means you're severely restricting your vitamin and nutrient intake, so you are advised to take vitamin supplements during this time, so you aren't missing out on anything vital.

There is a list of foods you can eat, and you have to stick to them to the letter. Oils and alcohols are also banned completely. You are restricting your calories, and you are eating high protein and low fat meals. In addition, you have to drink at least 2 litres of water every single day.

This is not a diet that you can pick up and put down. If you do it, you cannot repeat it again for two years. If you try it and quit before the 13 days are up, you have to wait six months before you can retry. This is to give your body time to recover.

Why Does It Work?

You really don't need to be a rocket scientist to figure out why this works. Limiting your calories by such a drastic amount is going to result in weight loss, but whether this is true weight loss, or water, is up for debate. The diet does claim that it can help to affect your metabolism over a longer-term period, through the effects of those 13 days. This could help you lose weight after this time, but it is likely that you will regain weight also.

Expected Weight Loss Results

If you manage to get to the end of the 13 days without quitting, your weight loss results are likely to be quite dramatic. The people behind the diet claim that you can lose up to 22lb in those 13 days, and that is a large amount to lose in such a fast amount of time. Again, it's unlikely to stay off, and this is a diet which is not sustainable, on medical grounds.

Example Meal Plans/Eating Suggestions

You might be wondering how you're supposed to get any nutrition at all in just 600 calories, and yes, it's a challenge. A sample daily meal plan could look something like this:

- Breakfast - A cup of coffee, you are allowed one cube of sugar
- Lunch - Two hard boiled eggs, one tomato, and cooked spinach (around 400g)
- Dinner - Steak (around 200g), with green salad, and dressing made with lemon and oil

The rest of the diet is very similar, although you can vary things up a little as you move through the 13 days, whilst sticking to the 600 calorie limit. It is best to look for sample meal plans which last for the entire diet's time if you are serious about sticking to this diet, to ensure that you get at least some nutritional value.

Warnings

Where do we start?

You've probably already grasped that this diet isn't really a recommended one, although it does give you results, which is the reason why we have included it as a fad diet you may consider. Anyone who has any health condition, concern, or is on any medication at all needs to speak to their doctor before considering this diet. You are also likely to be advised not to do it.

It is very likely that without the nutrients you need, you are going to suffer from side effects, and if you notice dizziness, confusion, or cramping of the muscles, you should stop the diet immediately and seek medical help.

Again, do not try this diet again until two years have passed, and if you gave up before the diet was over, give it six months until you attempt it once more.

Chapter 15: Military Diet

The Military Diet is currently one of the most popular around, mainly because of the large losses it promises. The diet is also quite easy to follow; however, you do have a set meal plan much of the time, which could result in boredom.

The diet is called the 'Military Diet' because those who designed the diet claimed that the military used it to get their soldiers into the best shape of their lives, however there is no direct or confirmed link to any army, so this should be taken with a pinch of salt.

What is the Military Diet?

The Military Diet is a restricted calorie diet which claims to help you lose up to 10lb in just one week. Of course, much of this weight is going to be water, and if you resume eating 'normally', the weight is likely to creep back on. Such is the life of a fad diet!

You might hear this diet called the '3 Day Diet', basically because you diet solidly for three days, with a less restrictive period after that. Your diet consists of three days of a set meal plan, which cannot be deviated from, and then four days off. You then repeat this cycle weekly, until you are happy with the amount of weight you have lost.

For the three days, you are following the seat meal plan, you cannot have any snacks in-between meals, and you are going to have around 1100-1400 calories per day. This is restricted because the recommended amount is 2000 for a woman, and 2500 for a man. This is the reason for the weight loss. For the other four days, you can eat more freely, but your choices should continue to be healthy; if you binge eat on 'bad' things during this time, you're going to make yourself sick, quite probably, and your metabolism isn't going to know what day it is. You should continue to have a low-calorie diet during those four days, although less so than the stricter three days.

Why Does It Work?

The diet works because of the low-calorie intake during the dieting three days, and the advice to remain as healthy as possible during the other days. By incorporating regular exercise and drinking plenty of water, the results can be quite large. Having said that, when you return to a regular eating pattern, e.g. you cut out those three restrictive days, you're going to put weight back on, even if you continue to eat as healthy as possible.

For a quick fix however, experts don't believe this diet is harmful per se, because the restricted period is quite short. Having said that, if you have any concerns, conditions, or you're on any medications, you know what to do - see your doctor first!

Expected Weight Loss Results

The diet designers claim you can lose up to 10lb in a week. Obviously, the exact amount may vary from person to person, and as soon as you begin to eat normally once more, you're likely to regain some of it, because much of what you're losing is water.

You can continue the diet cycle for as long as you want to, until you reach your ideal weight goal, provided you do not deviate from the three days of low calorie intake. Never attempt to extend this, as that is when the diet becomes potentially harmful.

Example Meal Plans/Eating Suggestions

The Military Diet has a set meal plan for the first three days, i.e. the three days during your dieting cycle. The rest of the time (four days) you can eat whatever you want, as long as you continue to make healthy choices, e.g. you don't go overboard with fatty foods, and you sick to lean meats, whole-grains, fruits, and vegetables etc. It is advised that your calorie intake is still low during those four days.

The three day plan is as follows:

Day 1
- Breakfast - 1 slice of toast with 2 tablespoons of peanut butter, and half a grapefruit. You can have a cup of tea or coffee if you want to (decaf)
- Lunch - 1 slice of toast with half a cup of tuna, and another cup of tea or coffee if you want to (decaf)
- Dinner - A cup of green beans with a 3oz serving of meat
- Dessert - A small apple, half a banana, and a cup of ice cream (vanilla)

Day 2
- Breakfast - 1 hard-boiled egg with 1 slice of toast and half a banana. A cup of tea or coffee if you want to (decaf)

- Lunch - 1 cup of cottage cheese, 5 saltine crackers, and 1 boiled egg. Again, a cup of tea or coffee if you choose to (decaf)
- Dinner - 2 hot dogs (no bread), half a cup of broccoli and half a cup of carrots
- Dessert - Half a cup of ice cream (vanilla)

Day 3
- Breakfast - 5 saltine crackers, a small apple, and a slice of cheddar cheese (1oz). A cup of tea or coffee if you want to (decaf)
- Lunch - 1 slice of toast and 1 egg (cooked to your choosing). You can have a cup of tea or coffee (decaf)
- Dinner - 1 cup of tuna
- Dessert - Half a banana with 1 cup of ice cream (vanilla)

Warnings

As with any diet, check things out with your doctor if you have any concerns at all. The Military Diet is a restrictive diet and very low in calories, but the restrictive phase is thought to be too short to be extremely dangerous. Having said that, a diet which restricts your calories to extreme amounts should always be approached with caution.

It is not the best idea to follow this diet for a long period of time, e.g. months without a break, because you are running the risk of a nutrient deficiency. The overall healthiness of this diet also relies upon you being heathy during your four days off too, with plenty of fruits and vegetables for good nutritional value.

Conclusion

And there we have it, 15 of the most common fad diets on the market. Of course, there are countless more obscure ones, and additional ones will come and go all the time. It's impossible to tell you about every single fad diet, but from this list, you should have a general idea of what these types of diets can help you achieve.

Some are healthier than others. For example, we didn't really talk up the Copenhagen Diet for a good reason - it's unhealthy, regardless of the extreme weight loss results. The health benefits of the Atkins Diet, the Keto Diet, and the South Beach Diet in particular are still up for debate, but if you can follow them correctly, incorporate them into a healthy lifestyle, and vary up your meals accordingly, you could find that you can lose weight, maintain it, and stay healthy in the process.

Fad diets are called that because they are not designed to be prolonged. Diets like the Keto Diet don't really fall into that strict category, because they're supposed to encourage lifestyle changes. Yo yo dieting is very unhealthy, and it plays havoc with your body and metabolism. Whilst you might want to lose weight for whatever reason, e.g. a wedding or a vacation, it is always better to attempt to reach your goal in a slower and more sustainable manner. By doing this, you learn about good and healthy food choices, and this ensures your body gets exactly what it needs, without restricting nutrients in any way.

Of course, most diets promise great results, but what you're actually seeing on the scales is a loss of water, at least at first. It is impossible to sustain a large weight loss for more than a couple of weeks, because it is going to inevitably plateau out. This is also because your body starts to think it's going to starve. Any change in your eating habits puts the red warning lights on, and your body thinks 'hang on a minute', putting into place plan B, to make sure it gets the nutrients it needs. Of course, this should level out over time, as your body realises that it's not starving, and that it overreacted a little, but in the short term, this can mean stubborn weight loss which doesn't seem to be moving not he scales. This is the number one reason why people lose hope and drop a diet, as well as cravings too.

If you're certain you want to go down the fad diet route for a short-term fix, the best idea is to find a diet which you can follow easily, which isn't going to confuse you, and one which you can make plenty of delicious meals from, according to your tastes. After you've achieved that you need to achieve, turn your attention to living a healthy life overall, with plenty of fruits, vegetables, whole-grains, lean proteins, and healthy fats. Throw in plenty of exercise and alcohol only in moderation, and you're looking at a sustainable weight, and a healthy life.

Good luck!

Please see other Titles from

ARYLA PUBLISHING

Children's Books
The Body Goo Series
The Billy Series
The Ruby Series
Emergency Service Series
Love Bugs & Animals Series

Adult Books
Self Help Books
Diet and Wellbeing
Comedy Books

FOR ALL
Coloring Books

Other Publications

<u>Eating My Feelings : Control Stress Eating</u>
By Fiona Welsh (Self Help)

Eat. Cry. Laugh. Repeat.

If you catch yourself

- **Chomping down on a box of donuts to celebrate the latest pay check.**
  - •
- **Draining a tub of ice cream after a fight with your significant other.**
  - •
- **Staring into an open refrigerator whenever you're bored.**

then you just might be an **Emotional Eater.**

Most people who are overweight use food as a comfort and coping mechanism; and are often unaware of the contributions of emotional eating to their waistlines. When diet is regulated by moods, emotional eaters will often try to 'self-medicate', by eating to get rid of unpleasant emotions, rather than when they feel hungry. And so, it is often the case that when feelings and food become linked, a food junkie is created, and the world becomes a little bit heavier. If this resonates with you, then the information inside this book is perfect for you.

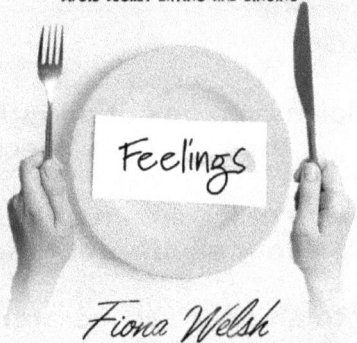

EATING MY FEELINGS

CONTROL STREET EATING WHEN HAPPY AND SAD,
AVOID SECRET EATING AND BINGING

Feelings

Fiona Welsh

Anxiety: Dealing With Anxiety & Panic Attacks –
By Fiona Welsh (Self Help)

Do you regularly feel like you are always worrying about something? Do you often feel fearful? Do you wake up with a sense of dread a lot of the time? Do you feel fine one minute and then you start overthinking, and your mind turns into a hamster wheel of 'what if' situations and scenarios? Do you feel generally uneasy a lot of the time, and you can't really pinpoint a reason why?

If you are nodding your head to most of the above then it could very well be that you are suffering from an anxiety disorder.

Anxiety is more common than you might even think. It is thought that 1 in every 13 people will suffer from an anxiety disorder at some stage in their lives, and this equates to around 7.3% of the world's population. The statistics are startling, and that makes anxiety the most common mental disorder in the spectrum.

If you're feeling like you might have a problem with anxiety, these statistics should give you a little hope – you're not alone, you're not going crazy, the world isn't the dark place that you might be led to believe; there is help at hand.

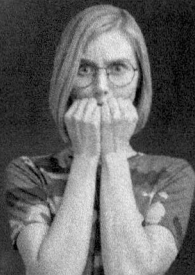

The Truth About Getting Old –
By Tyler Moses (Comedy)

Congratulations and welcome to the over 40s club! You have worked hard to get to this pinnacle point in life, so let's take a moment to celebrate being over 40 and everything that comes with it. Your body has been through a lot in order to get you over the hill, and your 40s is when some of your parts may start to, well, retire. During your time in the old person club, your body will experience new and not-so-exciting changes around every corner (even though we take corners slowly now as to avoid obstacles that may knock us off balance). Grab your Biotene and a large supply of antacids and sit back on your heating pad as we journey into the life of being over 40.

THE TRUTH ABOUT
GETTING
OLD

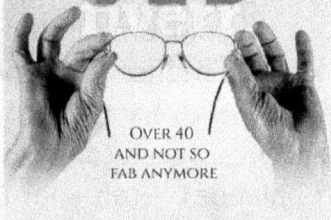

OVER 40
AND NOT SO
FAB ANYMORE

TYLER MSES

How to Make Money Online –
By Fiona Welsh (Self Help – Business)

Unfortunately, the pot of gold at the end of the rainbow is yet to be found, there doesn't seem to be a Leprechaun smiling at whoever manages to stumble upon this long-famed prize, and as for the money tree, well, it's still as elusive as ever.

From time to time, we all find money hard to come by, and no matter how hard we work, or how much we save, it's likely that there are things we want and need that we can't afford at the present time. Obviously, that doesn't mean that your money situation is going to be difficult all the time, because cash flow ebbs and flows (pardon the pun) as much as anything in life, but finding ways to help it along a little is always a good thing.

The internet has changed so much about our modern-day lives, it is quite hard to think of anything that we don't use an online connection for in some way or another. From booking holidays, doing our grocery shopping, meeting the new Mr or Mrs Right in our lives, or finding a new job, the Internet connects it all. So, taking that thought a little further, can the Internet help us to earn a little extra cash when our flow isn't, well, flowing as fast as we would like?

Of course, it can!

The Internet is a fantastic place to start, and the beauty of all of it is that you can do it from the comfort of your armchair!

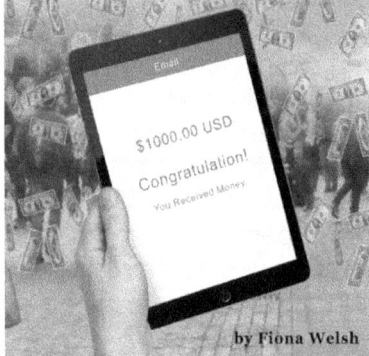

Keeping Your Children Safe –
By Fiona Welsh (Self Help – Business)

Without a doubt, the most important and treasured things we have in our lives are our children. We give birth to them, we raise them, we worry about them, and we love them to the end of the world and back again. It is no surprise that when we see worrying events on the news, it first makes us think of our children.

We can't protect our kids from everything in life, and we can't shield them from the things that are going on around the globe, but we can do our very best to keep them as safe as possible. As a parent you will no doubt be very familiar with the thought that you want to wrap your children up in cotton wool and avert their eyes from anything that isn't Disney magical. Things can and do happen, but part of the solution is to know how to teach your children about safety in general, in the right way. Learning to show them that it is fine to explore, fine to live, but that being on the lookout for danger is vital.

So, how do you do that? How do you tread that fine line between living life and avoiding dangerous situations?

KEEPING YOUR
CHILDREN
SAFE

INFORMATION AND ADVICE ON HOW TO PROTECT YOUR
CHILD AGAINST LIFE'S DARKER SIDE

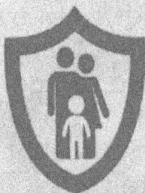

FIONA WELSH

We also have a selection of Adult Coloring Books to help relax pass the time and de-stress.
Beautiful Illustrations and puzzles in the back for your entertainment.

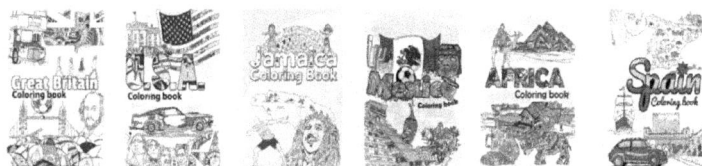

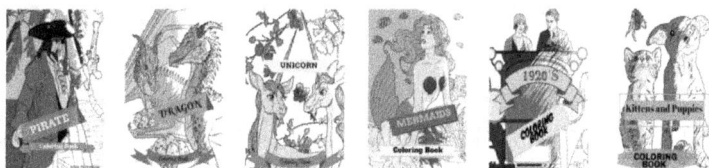

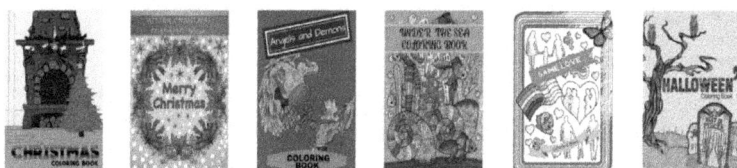

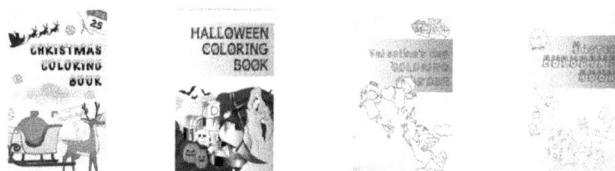

Visit **www.ArylaPublishing.com**
to find out about all new releases.

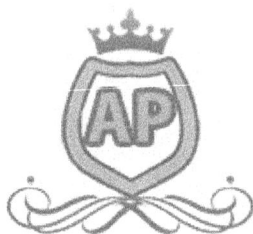

Follow us @arylapublishing on Twitter Instagram & Facebook

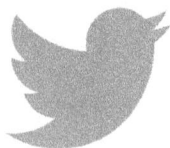

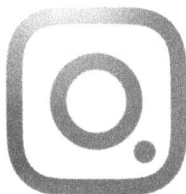

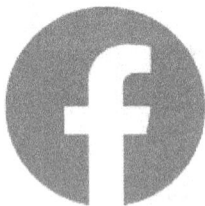

Search for Aryla Publishing on

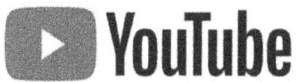

YouTube

Check out our _Book Trailers_

Subscribe **to keep up to date with new releases!**

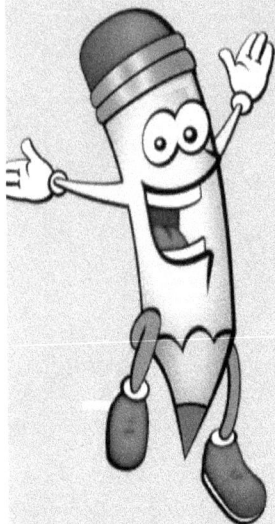

WE WOULD LOVE YOUR FEEDBACK

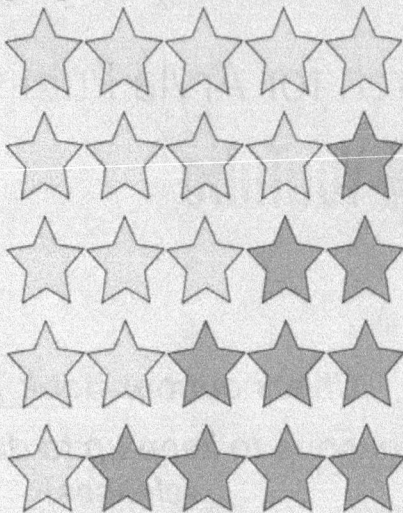

PLEASE LEAVE REVIEW AT:-
https://getbook.at/dietfads

www.ingramcontent.com/pod-product-compliance
Lightning Source LLC
Chambersburg PA
CBHW060516280326
41933CB00014B/2982

* 9 7 8 1 9 1 2 6 7 5 3 2 6 *